The
Words

By Sharon Milne Barbour

Welcome to our book *'The Magic of Words'*, you will find among these pages, positive vibration, wisdom, guidance and love for all of humanity.

There are verses of inspiring words that will resonate with each and every one of you in different ways. If you are holding this book in your hand, it is because you are the student as you travel your life's path and what you learn from these magical words you will one day teach to others.

Enjoy my friends, be inspired and most importantly find your true self and sparkle.

CONTENTS

	Acknowledgements	4
Section 1	**The inner wisdom of words**	7
	- Yin and yang	
Section 2	**Creating a magical life with words and your thoughts**	25
	- Heal yourselves	28
	- Awareness of self and the world around you	32
	- How to raise your vibration with thoughts and words	40
	- The 'I Am' moments	42
	- Thoughts can change your future	43

| Section 3 | **The guidance and wisdom words can hold** | 51 |

- 58 verses and writings of inspiration guidance and wisdom

| Section 4 | **Daily guidance messages for you** | 108 |

- 44 individual daily guidance teachings to help you move forward on your life's path

Notes and inspiration 152

We have included some blank pages for you to record your own positive thoughts and inspiration my friends.

About the author 171

The magic of words

Copyright © 2015 by Sharon Milne Barbour - Bengalrose Healing

Published by Bengalrose Healing

Author – Sharon Milne Barbour

Book cover illustration – by Zac Podilchuk and Sharon Milne Barbour

All rights are reserved. No part of this book may be reproduced by any mechanical, photographic, or electrical process, or in the form of a phonographic recording, nor may it be stored in a retrieval system, transmitted, or otherwise be copied for public or private use - other than for "fair use" as brief quotations embodied in articles. Reviews are not to be written without prior written knowledge of the publisher and author. The intent of the author is only to offer information of a general nature to help you on your spiritual path. In the event you use any of the information in the book for yourself, which is your right, the author and the publisher assumes no responsibility for your actions.

Section 1

The inner wisdom of words

Welcome to our book *'The Magic of Words'*, which we have written for all of mankind. We wish all future children of your world to be bought up in a vibration of love and positivity, and we feel their thoughts and words are key to this happening. Remember that mankind and any being in the universe, including other worlds, realms and dimensions, have a very powerful source at their grasp with the use of words and thoughts.

Words can determine how you develop on your life's path, as they are the base of your thought patterns. For example, when a child is born, the words you use to calm them, sing them to sleep and express your love, affects how that child will develop on its life path.

A child that is born into an environment of fear through dictatorships oppressing the people, unhappy relationships, abuse and poverty, means that child will grow up in an environment of neglect and be surrounded by words of fear. You see my friends, it's not just what the words are, it is the way the words are said, the intent and the tone within the voice.

The human mind and spirit has an amazing way of tuning into the vibration of the sound of the words that are spoken. It is the way the words vibrate out into the Universe that affects the human mind and the spirit within you.

So we are saying the children of your world will grow up in their environment of words in various languages, various meanings and various tones and vibrations. Their lives and their future will be moulded by the words that develop their thought patterns to survive in their environment.

As adults, my friends, take a look at yourselves and think about how you use your day-to-day language. Imagine you have just had something happen in your life – say, you have just created a wonderful painting, and when you show it to people, you listen to their words or silence. Some people will give you an excited, positive feedback straight away, others will hesitate before they share their thoughts; the latter will give you self-doubt about what you have achieved. Some might say positive words to you, but not in the same vibration as the excited first group of people. Then you will experience the ones that stay silent, and you will sense jealousy and contempt from them. You will also get the people that will openly criticize, and this could come from loved ones or a stranger.

Remember these are all words, even the silence holds silent words, which are your thoughts. These are all words said and meant in different ways which will affect how you react and feel about the situation, and how you move forward on your life's journey.

Now, this masterpiece you have created and the response you receive, will affect the outcome of how well you achieve in the future, and will affect how you respond to the words and vibration of words you have received. You might think it was a mistake to do this painting. The word 'mistake' is a negative; we would want you to think of it as an experience, which is a more positive word and way of looking at life, as we are all here to learn through experiences. How do you feel when you change the word 'mistake' to 'experience'? Do you see what we are saying? This is an experience in your life, this is an opportunity for you to reflect on what has been said and the words that were used. Remember, all true artists are never satisfied with what they achieve as they strive for that perfection in their work.

This applies to all arts, writers, landscapers, architects; anybody in your world who has a creative idea is never, ever fully satisfied with what they achieve. We see this as a wonderful thing for you, because you can do better, my friends, you can always strive to do better in life.

Every word that is spoken by you and your fellow mankind will affect you every second of your earth day. So we ask you to sit and look at the words you use on a day-to-day basis. The Universe is made up of energy, your world is made up of energy, you are made up of energy, the words that come out of your mouths are energy and the thoughts that vibrate from your mind are energy. THINK - all of this energy surrounds every single word that comes out of your mouth. As we have already said, it's not just the word that's used, it's also the tone and intent behind the spoken word that vibrates out to others.

The intent that affects the tone of the word should come from the heart and your inner spirit, with no malice or cruel intent. We see in the human form and with your ego how this can be hard to achieve. You cannot really disguise how you feel to your fellow man; they will always know within their inner spirit and in their heart if you have doubt in them, or do not believe in them. Your words change your energy around yourself and around the person you are speaking to. The empaths amongst you, who are more sensitive and tuned into the universe more, will understand this and be more aware of it.

So what do you think this means, my friends, this vibration that goes out into the universe? Think of the batteries you use to give energy to objects in your world. Think of the PLUS and MINUS signs, think of the negative words, the words of doubt; these are the minus energy words, and the positive words are the plus signs, both travelling out on energy wave vibrations into the universe. These PLUS and MINUS energies will attract the same energies back to them. Minus attracts minus, and plus attracts plus – and this will be how you live your life. If you keep using negative words, words of fear and doubt, words of not true meaning to you, this is the energy you will attract back into your life, so to lift your vibration you need to change the way you think and speak. The plus energy signs will go out into the universe, which will draw the plus energy signs back into your own energy field; this is what you want to achieve, and this is what you need for your life's path on earth. You will then be the person you are supposed to be and live your life as you should. You will also to be true to yourself and others in what you speak, and think and feel in a loving and kind way.

This can be hard for mankind, as you have been programmed for thousands of years to live in a controlled way, especially in the eastern world, and the parts of your world under dictatorships that control their societies through fear. Even in your Western world, you are controlled by your leaders and what your media choose to let you know. So you see this is a massive ask for mankind, to change the way you use your words and their vibrations, but it is achievable for you all, it is certainly very achievable for you all of humanity.

You must look at your words, see that they can be **magical** and so important to your everyday life. It's not just how you speak my friends, it is also the expression of your whole body, your energy field. Those amongst you that do not have speech through a physical impairment, will use their facial expression and body as a language to express how they feel, have you ever watched someone signing for the deaf, no words, look at their whole body and face and you will understand what we mean.

When someone speaks to you, look at their eyes; they express so many emotions, they show love or fear, shining their inner energy through to you. It is very interesting for us to observe mankind and how your body expresses these feelings, but every day, a lot of mankind is not aware of this, and you take it all for granted, my friends. But if you just sat and observed your world around you, you would see it differently. For example, try sitting in a café one day and just watch people; see how they interact, observe the love, the fear, the sustainment amongst mankind – just observe, and you will see what we mean.

To help with the example of the words we were talking about, the PLUS and the MINUS energies, we have placed some words in this chapter for you, replacing the negative words with positive words which you can use in your day-to-day lives to lift your vibration and positive way of being.

You have to reset your brain from the **minus** setting to the **plus** setting, and when you do this, my friends, a whole new way of being will open up to you. You will be raised up onto a higher energy pattern, drawing in positive energy and thoughts. Your persona will alter, you will feel lighter, happier and more in tune with yourself, and this will alter the world around you. Others will be drawn to your uplifted vibration; you will also find that the people around you that live on the minus battery wavelength vibration will become more distant to you and the people on the plus battery wavelength will be drawn to you. It is natural for this to happen for your progression and ascension on your life's journey. Some of these negative people could be family or friends. This does not mean they will be out of your life, it means they will be held at your positive boundary so that their negative words, fear and critics will not affect you, and the plusses will be drawn into your energy bubble and raise your vibration further – just as you will raise theirs.

There are a lot of lists in your world showing negative and positive words on your internet and in your books, but this is our list, our take on words, and the use of feelings and tones you use in your daily lives. If you use and live by the **PLUS energy** words your world will be a different place to live in, my friends. You could all learn to live in this positive way, and the start of this is through your thought pattern; even a small change every day will make a difference.

We see in the light workers that have chosen to work with spirit and be an advocate for spirit, cringe at the words and the way they used to speak before seeing this positive, loving way of being. They have adapted and changed as the light has come in, and they have understood the love of spirit and the way we are. They understand the human form can exist and be like we are in the spirit realm.

So take the first step, my friend, and change your thought pattern today. Which are you? **Minus** or **Plus**?

MINUS energy	**PLUS energy**
Hate	Love
Miserable	Happy
Dark	Light

Obstacle	Experience
Grief	Acceptance
Cry	Laugh
Cruel	Kind
Dictatorship	Freedom
Rough	Smooth
Lost	Found
Dark	Light
Negative	Positive
Mistake	Lesson
Die	Live
Punish	Forgive
Frown	Smile
Sick	Well
Distance	Near
Selfish	Share
Shut	Open

Nothing	Plenty
Silence	Speak
Degrade	Uplift
Jail	Sanctuary
Deflate	Inspire
Hit	Hug
Sly	Honest
Deceit	Transparency
Disconnect	Connect
Broken	Whole
Mist	Clear
Nothing	Universe
Addiction	Clean
Fake	Real
Lie	Truth
Take	Give
Despair	Elevation

Distraught   Euphoric

Depressed   Happy

Ugly   Beautiful

Unperceptive   Insight

Yin and yang

Have you heard of Yin and Yang, my friends? The words come from the Chinese philosophy and religion on your earth, for the two principles, Yin for negative and dark, and Yang positive and bright; the belief is that those different energy interactions influence the destinies of living beings, creatures and other things in your world. We feel that the Yin and Yang example from the Chinese society on earth has a good basic understanding of creating oneness amongst humans. It's simple message is the distinctions between good and bad, for instance shadow cannot exist without light and good words counteract negative energy as they have a more positive energy vibration. So are the Chinese simply saying there cannot be light without dark? In the sense of nature and the sun casting shadows, then yes. But amongst humans, there can be just light, shining from within you, without any darkness – and the magic use of positive words can help with this.

Yes, your human form will always cast a shadow from the earth's sun, but if you ascend into a kinder, more loving way of being, in thinking and speaking you will only ever admit the divine light and love to your fellow humans from the spirit within. Every positive word, thought and connection to spirit and the divine helps your inner spirit grow, enveloping you in its love, wisdom and knowledge. Love is key to sweeping away the darkness (Yin) within your human essence and world.

The more of you who recognise this and change, the more love and light can shine through the dark cracks of your world; have faith that one day all the dark cracks will disappear, and only love and light will shine on earth.

As you change your use of words and way of thinking into this positive way of being, you will become more open to others' feelings as well as your own. Your intuition will step up a gear or two; listen to this intuition, as it is a gift from us. As you open up more spiritually, we will also be able to guide thoughts of love, kindness and wisdom into your mind to help with your words, and we will give you the gut feelings to follow and thoughts to act on. This intuition comes from your spirit within as we try to guide you, which is why we say it is a gift from us.

Your thoughts and way of thinking are what you need to change to speak the positive words needed to improve your life and way of being. We thought we would lay out some examples for you of language use, to help you raise your vibration in your speech and thought patterns; the negative words or thoughts are highlighted in bold for you.

Example 1:

Minus energy:

"**No,** I did not tell him, he looked **so miserable** when I saw him so I did not speak to him, **I'll let him get on with it** and tell him my news the next time I see him."

Plus energy:

"I did see him but he did not seem his normal self today, so I felt it was not the right time to say anything. I hope he's all right, I'll ring him later to check he's ok."

A simple sentence example for you, this is more about the tone as well as the odd word like miserable *that would bring in the negative energy and thoughts. The second one has a kinder, more compassionate tone, expressing consideration and love, as the speaker wants to contact them to see they are all right. Always follow through these kind actions you state to others, as the feeling you need to contact someone is often guidance from us.*

Example 2:

Minus energy:

"I know you are concerned **BUT** I need more time in my days and **if I carry on like this I will burn myself out, oh why do all these things keep happening to me? I'm so fed up, I never have time for me** and everybody wants **a piece of me at the moment.**"

Plus energy:

"Thanks for your concern. Ok, I know I have so much to do, so I am going to look at my schedule and see what can wait, plan my days better and ask for help when needed. This will help me manage my time better, so I'm more productive, and free up time outside work to spent more time with loved ones and friends. Then I can have time to concentrate on planning to achieve my goals too, and give me more time for myself as well.

In this example the lady was being gently reminded by her friend that she was overdoing it on a daily basis, family and friends were demanding a lot of her, and she needed to take control of her own life and actions, as it was affecting her work and home life. In the first statement she feels sorry for herself and is blaming the world around her for her circumstances.

In the second response, she is someone who has changed her thought patterns, realising she needs to change her way of thinking, and you can see the more positive thought pattern that will draw in better energy. She has decided to take personal responsibility and make priorities, take ownership of herself and quite importantly, ask for help to achieve this time management in her life. It is important you are happy in yourself and achieve your own goals, then you will be at your best for your loved ones in your life.

Example 3:

The magic of words

Joan is having a conversation with her friend about a job interview:

Minus energy

" **Aw, I've** got my interview on Friday, I'm **not looking forward to it**, I **hope** I get this job, **not sure I have the right qualifications though**, and **my last interview was so bad.**"

Plus energy:

"I am really looking forward to my interview on Friday. I feel very positive about the job, I have so much I can contribute to the company. I know I can do this role as I can see myself in this job. I'll ring you on Friday and let you know how I get on."

You can see in the minus sample the negativity as she puts herself down and has self-doubt; she's putting out to the universe that she is not good enough and won't get the job. This is how she will come across on the day, too. It's a self-fulfilling prophecy. Now, after reading the second speech, you can see the more uplifted feeling in the voice and thoughts of the Plus energy. Remember, when you are in this type of situation, it helps the energies if you visualise being in this job role as if you are living it.

These three basic examples are just to make you think about how you respond by thoughts and words to every situation in your lives.

STOP and **Think** before you speak, think of it like learning to put on a safety belt for every car trip you take; you will get into the habit and as the energy shifts to the positive way of being, it will become second nature to you.

This is an assured safety mechanism for your future ascension into PLUS energy, and a love and light existence.

Section 2

Creating a magical life with words and your thoughts

Many of you on earth are starting to understand the negative and positive energies, the minus and plus signs, especially those of you who are light workers.

We see a lot of you still doubt and question these theories and that they can help mankind move forward. The only thing that stops this negative/positive theory working is you, with the fears, anxieties and illusions you create in your minds about the world you live in. This holds you back on your life's path, keeping you in the negative energy streams.

To move forward, my friends, you need to resolve these issues within your human essence, and allow the energy to flow freely around your body. This will allow the positive energy to become strong in the love and light, and the negative energies to fade.

You do all create a path before you come to a physical existence in the universe,; at this time, yours is to be on earth. The path is mapped out for you and we hold the blueprint in the spirit realm, so we can guide you and the spirit within on your life's journey. We are aware of events that might affect your life's path and knock you off-course a bit, but as we have said in our previous books, we cannot be one hundred per cent on this. There will be things that come onto your pathway we had not anticipated, but we deal with this as it happens from the spirit realm, helping your spirit within to get back on track.

The ones that doubt this negative and positive energy theory, and the creation of a reality through affirmations, manifestations, thoughts and words to help mankind move forward, believe that some humans are so broken within, through traumas within their physical human life, that they cannot be helped by this theory.

We do see when humans hurt each other how it affects the human essence, and it takes a great deal of healing. While you are in the third dimension, sometimes the healing is needed from the medical professions on earth, as well as the spiritual realm encouraging the positive way of being. As you ascend into your fourth dimension, the healing will become more from your human mind, the spirit within healing you without your medical nurses and doctors. This is because as you move into the fourth dimension, the harm humans cause each other through abuse and the crimes against humanity will decrease, and there will not be so many broken humans in your world crying out with pain and fear because of what their lives have brought to them. Your minds will start to reset themselves, bringing clarity and greater understanding to the human race.

As you ascend into the fifth dimension have faith, my friends, that humanity will heal itself, there will be no sickness of the body or mind and no medicines will be needed. The world will be a different place to what you know it as today. There will no longer be fear, anxiety and hate amongst mankind to cause harm to other humans.

So, my friends, you can see the picture we are trying to show you with our words, which is just to have faith and trust in what we are saying about creating your own life and changing into a positive way of being.

NOW, have you ever thought why you should not have a life full of abundance, health and wealth, a nice house and nice cars? You can still be a beautiful person within, being kind and helping others in your world, and you can bring in an abundance of love and wealth through the positive energy, thoughts, words and affirmations we have been talking about.

Now, this positive pure energy from the love and light of the spirit realm and universe will be drawn to those of you who have a positive attitude with pure heart and good intentions. Those of you that choose to manifest and pretend to be in the love and light will draw in more negative energies, and will struggle to universe and spirit realm know the true intent that lies within you, not the outside façade you are putting on; this is what the universe can sense, and that is what you will receive back to your energies. Those that draw in these negative energies will have problems with ill health, regret and strife in life, and they will not heal their fears and concerns, so remember the PLUS and MINUS energies.

Heal yourselves

We see on your earth a world of too much sickness, pain and too much fear, my friends. The fears are survival-based for example - Where is the next meal coming from? How can we afford these medical bills? Who's going to help us? Why is this happening to us?

Can you see the negative energies in this fear by these words alone?

We know that mankind can heal themselves through positive thoughts and energy, because you see it in simple terms when you become ill through the stress of your lives. In the western world it's more to do with your pace of life that causes anxiety and stress. In other areas of the world it can be nature, manmade situations in war-torn countries, religious differences and stress that these situations cause. All of this is surrounded by the minus negative energy you absorb, which then manifests in the body. You can imagine that where there is poor diet and inhumane treatment, the poor humans caught up in this situation struggle to find any positive energies. This is where the rest of mankind can come in and help each other, and bring the PLUS energies to these people.

When humans become sick, including with the terminal illnesses amongst mankind, humans worry and fear and think, why me? We see this as natural for you, after thousands of years of this way thinking, BUT it is time to reboot your brains, and discard this negative way of thinking. When you are sick you draw more negative energies into your body, and the sickness within you collects it and feeds off it, making the symptoms worse. Have you noticed that when you are stressed or have high anxiety, any ailment you suffer with increases? This is because the minus energy targets the weak areas of your body and mind. You need to build up the positive energy and direct it to flow round these weaker areas to protect them and let them heal.

Now for those of you who have lost loved ones to sickness on your earth, it is hard for you to understand this as you have seen the pain they have suffered, and the pain that reflects around the surviving loved ones and friends. BUT do TRUST, my friends, that you can heal yourselves and humanity. If you could all from the moment you are born, be taught to think in the positive vein: *'I am well, balanced and positive',* this would bring the Mother Earth back to a balanced energy again and humanity will not suffer the illnesses, the anguish and the fear it suffers now.

Around your world, there are healers amongst you who are starting to understand this and spread the word to others. Some of these healers have healed themselves, even from your diseases and mental illnesses, with this positive way of thinking and trusting in the divine for help with this.

We know you understand by now the third dimension energy that you exist in at the moment, and as more and more of you start to think in the positive energy, changing your thought pattern and your words, you will ascend into the fourth dimension energy. It's as simple as saying when you wake up every day, 'I am well, and I am balanced.' If a doctor tells you, you have something wrong, or you develop a viral illness, visualise yourself without it and visualise yourself well, and ask for healing from your angels and guides of pure love and light energy. Remember the negative MINUS energy is attracted to you when you are ill, as your mindset goes into a negative way of thinking and your mind and energy field can be clouded if you have pain with your illness or health condition.

Now, you also need to ask yourself, why did I get this condition or illness? Was it through unhealthy eating and no exercise, or is it from the stress that's in my life? You need to sort out in your own lives the stress, fears and anxieties that lie within you from the traumas you have experienced on your human path while on earth. It is easy for us to say this, but we do see the humans who have not yet seen our light and do not understand the love that comes from spirit, and struggle with this new way of thinking we wish for all of humanity.

We have put this into words hoping all who read this will start to understand that every bit of positive energy and light that comes into your world will move you all into a better way of being. Have TRUST, my friends, that future generations will exist in the way we are saying, with the Positive PLUS energy vein, in a balanced, well-being and self-healing existence. The human mind will become more powerful in the PLUS energy, because it's you, your own mind, your thoughts and words that are going to cure you, with the link to your healers in the spirit realm.

Awareness of self and the world around you

We also feel it is key to healing and lifting your energy vibration that each one of mankind has greater self-awareness of their own body and spirit within. As you develop this awareness of self, you will bring this out into the world about you. One thing that will help with this is to bring **Mindfulness** into your lives. We are sure this is a word you would recognise but not fully understand as yet, unless you practice it.

In the spirit world, we have great knowledge of mindfulness and being aware of the moment, but we don't have time as you know it in your limited third dimension energy. We live in the fifth dimension energy where we do not follow a time-constrained existence; this helps to give us great awareness and clarity of everything around us. Our thought stream is telepathic by nature, and we have great control over our mind links and when we connect. We are aware of what's gone before us and what's to come, but we don't let these thoughts or words affect our energy or the decisions we take. We are also very aware of our realm and the uniqueness that everything within it holds.

We have been encouraging the mindfulness practice among humans for centuries – look at some of your Eastern countries for the history of this. In your western world it is becoming a welcome trend at the moment, as the light builds and more and more light workers are teaching this and making others aware.

We know this is a positive way forward for mankind to help you connect more with yourself, the world around you and other humans. Learning and understanding mindfulness will also aid you in meditation which helps to de-stress you, clearing and raising your energies to aid ascension.

The benefits of mindfulness help in these ways:

- It cultivates more awareness and stabilises the mind

- You become clear-seeing (have clarity) in everything around you and within yourself

- It changes your perspective on your world and your thought patterns

- It brings wisdom, as you see your world differently

- It helps de-stress you by casting worrying thoughts to the side and giving your busy mind a rest.

Humans dwell too much on their past thoughts, fears and anxieties, and you then bring these fears and old habits into your thoughts for your future. You are all so busy in this 3D energy stream that's limiting you, you miss the single unique moment you are passing through.

Your minds are amazing things, my friends, with great power that could unfold great things for mankind. At the moment your minds are restricted by dwelling on your past memories and emotions, which then influence how you look at your future. Your mind is judgmental and creates its own misperceptions of situations and the world around you.

Your mind connects to your senses – sight, hearing, touch, smell and taste. We see you see without seeing, hear without hearing, touch without touching, smell without smelling and taste without truly tasting. You also have another sense, **Knowing**, which is like a sixth sense and is in your mind field and your energy field. What do we mean? Knowing is something that you use without realising it, but it is a weak sense at the moment in most of mankind. When tapped into and strengthened, this ability will bring you knowledge from the universe, clarity to your thinking, wisdom and greater understanding. To enhance this in the human form you need to master mindfulness – raising your **awareness**, and changing your mindset regarding how you look at the world around you. Once you do this, you will shift to the Plus energy stream, enhancing all your senses, including the ability to see and sense clearly in your lives. Working with this alongside the positive words and intentions behind those words, and mankind will start to shift toward reaching their full potential.

You rush along in your world, thinking you are aware of the world around you, but you are not. The simplest way for us to describe this in words is to give an example: you are given ten red pencils laid out next to each other in a row; most people will think they are all the same and not take a second look at them; as long as they function and serve the purpose that is all that matters. BUT each pencil is unique! If you stopped and looked at each individual pencil, you would be able to describe each one and the uniqueness that makes them different from each other. As you did this you would be more aware of that moment in time, as if you have slowed down time to stop and become aware of these 10 red pencils. You can feel them, look at them all over, smell them, listen to them and even taste them. When you are this aware you are being **mindful,** and this is what mindfulness means.

We do laugh though – we say be more aware, but if you followed this example of the red pencils to everything in your day, you would not get much done! BUT do you see what we are saying?

To help you on the path of mindfulness we are going to give you a couple of simple exercises to get you started. But we recommend you find a good meditation teacher to guide you.

Breathing exercise

Shut your eyes

o Now concentrate your attention on your breath, your normal everyday breathing pattern. The breath will be center stage of your awareness, just let your body breathe for itself as we do every day.

o Take your awareness to the gentle flowing of the IN and OUT breath, notice how it feels travelling up and down your airways to your lungs. How does it feel in your nostrils, and then as your breath flows to your lungs?

o Feel the breath leaving the body and re-entering. Where do you feel the sensations? In the nostrils, mouth, stomach? Relax and just ride the waves of your breathing moment by moment, with each breath.

- Remind yourself of the attention you need to give this, concentrating on the breathing.

- Can you smell the breath, is there any taste, are there sensations in your mouth?

- Imagine the breath flowing out. Does it have colour, or is there any moisture?

- If any past and present thoughts intrude, just gently and lovingly let the thoughts pass by, re-establishing focus on the breath. Refocus as earlier on the nostrils, lungs and stomach.

- Now expand your awareness to your whole body. How does the breath feel? Your skin breathes – can you feel this and take note of any sensations you pick up on?

- Now take yourself back to focusing on the nostrils, the breath coming in and out of the body. Just rest on these feelings, being in the moment, and when you feel ready, go back to normal activities.

This is a simple everyday exercise for you to use, to help bring clarity and rest to your busy mind. The more you practice this the better it will be, and you will be able to do it for longer periods when your third dimension busy energy life allows.

Glass of water exercise

- Sit in a chair near a table and place by you a glass of water.

- When you are ready, pick up the glass of water and hold it in both hands. Hold the glass in front of your face so you can clearly see it with your eyes. Examine the glass and see what you observe. Is it smooth, is it rough, is it dull, is it chunky, is the glass thin or thick, are there any scratches on it, and are there colours?

- Now notice the temperature of the glass.

- Now move the glass carefully around to one of your ears and gently rotate it in your hand. Do you notice any sound?

- Now take the glass and lift it to your mouth, but before you swallow any water, smell the glass and notice any odours. Also take notice of how your mouth feels inside – is it dry, is there any saliva?

- Now swallow some of the water. How does

the water feel? Is it smooth, is it cold, is it warm, what does it taste like and does it cause sensations in your mouth?

o Now imagine following the water from the mouth to your stomach, seeing it on its journey inside you. Notice any sensations.

o When you feel ready, set the glass back on the table and reflect on your experience.

This second simple exercise again really takes your awareness to the uniqueness of the glass of water, something you all take for granted every day.

I now feel you are beginning to understand where we are coming from on the ideas of mindfulness and raising your awareness. Practice regularly, my friends, and see where it takes you.

How to raise your vibration with thoughts and words

As we have mentioned, a good way to start to change your energy into a more positive vein is through affirmative words with good intent behind them. We thought we would give you some examples that are used in our friend's Bengalrose teachings today. We will start with affirmations; these are great ways for you to send the energy out to us and the universe, on the PLUS energy wave.

Love and kindness affirmation example

"During my day may I be happy, healthy, free from conflict, drama, negativity and all mental, physical and financial restraints. Instead, may I be blessed in abundance of kindness, positive energy, happiness, wealth, and peace and love. May I give and receive sincere acts of love and kindness throughout my day. "

This is an affirmation you can do daily. As well as raising your own energies, it also helps to raise the energies of others around you. It's best to sit in the silence and close your eyes, and take yourself to your inner being, then repeat the words once in your head, believing in yourself and what you are saying.

Now, I want you to think of a close friend, family member or pet and send them these healing, positive thoughts.

Next, send them to someone you know but not very well – a neighbour, for example.

Lastly, send them to someone you struggle to get on with, or feel you have conflict with in day-to-day life.

You will be amazed by how your energies will change; sending the love to someone you have conflict with in your own mind will help diffuse this negative energy and enable you to move forward and past it. Are you starting to see how all this can help you, my friends?

Now we introduce the **'I am'** affirmations, to become aware of self and raise your energies.

The 'I Am' moments

The **'I Am'** moment is key to you lifting your energies; remember this all starts with you. We suggest you do a meditation mantra for five minutes each day, repeating the chosen affirmation to reinforce the positive energy vein in your lives. We have listed a few below for you to try:

I am Love and joy

I am happy

I celebrate me!

I am willing to let go

I choose love

Love and peace

I release my stress

I am the best I can be

My mind is at ease

I deserve to be happy

I am beautiful

I am loved

I love and respect myself

I am strong and powerful

I am calm

I am at peace

To do the mantra, sit in a quiet space where you will not be disturbed. Take a few deep, cleansing breaths then go to normal breathing, and repeat in your mind or out loud the chosen mantra words. A good method is to get into a smooth breathing pattern, with the words being said on the outward breath. If your mind wanders, just observe the thought, let it pass by and go back to repeating the mantra. The more you practice, the easier this will become for you.

Thoughts can change your future

"You live in a very busy society trudging along accepting your lot."

Not a positive statement is it?

But a lot of you live in this mindset. You might feel you accept your life as it is as you are not worthy of more, and you accept your lot because that's the way it is. You have lost confidence in yourselves and the universe to make changes – *"I have tried and they don't happen, so why bother?"* is the attitude.

Remember we want the best for you, and the words and kind intention of this book will help you unlock your mind, raise your awareness levels, and draw in the positive energy you need to ascend on your life's path. We will also help you manifest things in your life for the better, so you will be lifted into a positive place. But like all things in your life, nothing is handed to you on a plate, and you have to work at it.

You were given the magic talent of imagination. When you create what you desire on paper in the form of positive words with kind, loving intent, with no detriment to others to help manifest your dreams, you can then take it to the magic land of imagination and imagine you are living it. This seeps into your conscious and subconscious mind, and then it helps you create a reality of energy that the Universe can bring back to you. WOW – is that not amazing?!

Beware of how you write your affirmations, and the intent behind them in your thoughts. We advise all are done under prayer in the divine love and light, so you start off in your positive energy mindset.

We have laid out two examples. In A, this reveals doubt that the person saying it will still achieve their wishes and goals. Example B is from the heart, and the imagination *'you are living them.'* Please read both out loud and see how you feel, as more positive energy is being reflected out when you say example B.

Example A

Divine forever loving spirit, I see a future of health and wellbeing for my family and friends.

I see a future of no money worries and peace within our lives. We will be mortgage free, moving within two years to a lovely three-bedroom, house, garage and garden in the Surrey area.

My Husband will have some permanent freelance work for 2-3 days a week and the other days perusing his new businesses – he is well and happy.

My healing business will grow and my spiritual path with it, serving you the best I can.

My two sons will be happy, living fulfilling, healthy and strong lives.

My grandchild is well, loved and happy.

We will have a VW camper van to take me, my husband and the dogs off to the sea for breaks.

My friends will be healthy and true.

I can serve you the best I can at all times.

Example B

Divine forever loving spirit, I have health and wellbeing for my family and friends.

I have no money worries and peace within our lives. We are mortgage free, living in a lovely three-bedroom house, garage and garden in the Surrey area.

Chris has some permanent freelance work for

2-3 days a week and the other days perusing his new businesses – he is well and happy.

My healing business has grown and my spiritual path with it, serving you the best I can.

My two sons are happy, living fulfilling, healthy and strong lives.

My grandchild is well, loved and happy.

We have lovely holidays that keep us relaxed and well in our camper van.

My friends are healthy and true.

I serve you the best I can at all times.

You can see in B that the person uses her imagination to imagine living the existence she wanted. Notice the removal of the words *can, see, will*, replaced with the word *have, has, are* – the doubt has been taken away. These might seem subtle changes, my friends, but MY, don't they make a difference.

What to be aware of when creating your dreams.

During your manifestation creating, stay aware of these important four points:

First, don't try too hard to make things happen. Lose the fear you won't receive, just TRUST. The underlying emotion of fear is a prayer that asks for the experience not to happen. When you have a strong emotion that differs from what you are visualising, your emotions are the more powerful request that the Universe hears. So, ask your angels to help you align your heart and your head during your visualisations.

Your verse will be a statement to the universe, based on trust that expects to receive it. Once you get a feeling of peace in you and a certainty of the inevitability of your manifestation, stop asking for it. Instead, shift your energy to expecting it to happen. Imagine you are living that existence

Second, be sure to release your request completely. So often, we hang onto our desires and don't surrender them fully to the universe. So it is important your verse is correct and has everything in it you wish for. But be realistic within the boundaries of your life. Example: "Please bring me a diamond studded car and mansion in the Bahamas." It sounds wonderful, but how will you maintain this new life style? You could end up on your own, because no-one else was mentioned. Food for thought …

Third, allow time for things to happen; your angels and guides are dealing with mankind's free will, and they have to go off to make sure that what's needed is in place for you. On your path, you will receive what is in the best interests of you and those around you. It is good to add to all your affirmations: *'with the best outcome for myself and others'* – as we are all intertwined. Ask your angels and guides for guidance on this, as they are here to help you.

You do all come down here with a life plan to live your life to its full potential, moving towards the light path your inner spirit and we desire for you. This moment in time, and reading this book, is part of your path, it is no accident, my friends. Think of your angels and guides as team mates – they are here to work with you. Your intentions create your experiences, so ask us to help you align your intentions with love, and you'll experience the love that truly surrounds you, when you all work as a team.

Fourth, the angels and guides need a clear message from you. Stay motivated, as you will also have to work to help create your dreams, and it will not be instant. If you have asked, for example, *"I want to be thinner"*, you could become ill and become thinner that way. Be specific. *"Please help me become slimmer in a healthy way."* Or instead of: *"I would like lots of money and a big house"*, try saying: *"Please help me have no money worries with no detriment to others, my family are safe and healthy, and their future is secure."* You can give a time-frame to this, but be realistic.

We would like to end this chapter with a reminder you are students here to learn on earth, but also teachers. It is key for mankind that your children of the earth are raised in the love and light PLUS positive energy vibration. This book will give you the basic education you need to this and inspire you to follow this path, to love wisdom and the divine. Be **Inspired,** my friends, and be the **Inspirer**.

Section 3

The guidance and wisdom words can hold

We know you will enjoy these inspiring words, which are full of wisdom and guidance for you all. Please speak these words to inspire others.

The spirit from within

Your human essence joins with your divine spirit, both working together to create a unique being.

You link at the moment of conceptions innocence, a spark of the divine pure in love and light.

You both work tirelessly together to full fill your life's path; you all have a mission and a message to be sent out to others.

The separation of your spirits is planned when you return home; loved ones left behind then miss the physical presence.

They also miss your heavenly spirit, as this was your soul, the essence of you, and your true self that shone out to others.

There is great joy when you all reunite in the divine home source, the source of love and light, true knowing and knowledge.

You will wrap your love around each other again my friends when you all meet to carry on your spirit paths together.

The universe is yours, go out into the endless space and search for the wisdom and knowledge you seek.

Faith

Faith comes from with-in you. Have faith in your own abilities and the rest will follow.

Smile

Smile as you have never smiled before in the mirror, then look at your reflection beaming back at you. This is how others will see you, when you smile a beam of light shines in their world.

Have a vision

Your vision
is our vision,
live it,
breath it,
we will be part of it.

Intuition

Hesitation causes uncertainty, uncertainty affects your confidence, and lack of confidence affects your self-esteem.

Don't hesitate in life, have confidence and follow your intuition, it is a good friend to you; believe in and trust it, as it is a gift that comes from us.

Abundance

Abundance comes from within, it is your kindness, love and true self.

Abundance is your family, friends and animals in your life.

Abundance is being safe, warm and nourished.

Abundance is security, health and shelter.

Abundance is you as a whole and all the goodness around you.

When you have abundance give it out to those that don't.

Live in love and light and you will have abundance.

A fragile world

People are fragile, even those that seem to shine.

Be careful how you treat each other my friends, some of you keep your cracks well hidden.

Shine out love and light and heal your friends and family so the cracks you all carry can heal.

You and the world will be whole again.

Explore

Don't be afraid to explore new possibilities' in your life's, they are what will make you grow.

Energy

Every day you will witness positive and negative energy around you. Live in the positive energy, yes beware of the negative in your world, but don't let it stop you moving forward in love and light energy in your life.

Be true to yourself

Look at others, as you would wish them to look upon you, their eyes will always tell the truth as will your eyes. Always be true to yourself and others; see them through their eyes deep into their souls, then trust your intuition.

Look beyond

Time is the essence of your existence, look beyond time to find your true self.

You

You are awesome
You are you
You let your light shine
You will be strong
You will be wise
You will learn from hurt
You will heal from harm
You know who you are
You need to be you
You are awesome

Look within

Confirmation of who you are, is deep within you.

Find yourself to find the confirmation you seek.

To be you, be happy and follow your passions in life.

Move away from harm and those that do not love you.

You will then find yourself and all the confirmation you need.

Light up the world

Light up the world with your smile.

This will reflect in others like a mirror.

Smiling and laughter is contagious, be the person that spreads it and all will smile with you.

Smile and laugh your way through life and light up your world.

Gather near

Hold out your arms and gather your loved ones near.

They will give you strength my friends.

They are your inspiration, your listeners and your support network.

Their love is your love.

Your light is their light.

Blend and be as one, you will know peace.

Spark of life

A spark, a light in the dark

A glimpse of hope

The light casts a shadow

The shadow stretches before you

Always beside you

You are the light

We are the shadow

Even in the dark

Our shadow is with you

Light your spark to see us

Hear us and feel us

Sparkle and shine bright

Healing

Healing is forgiveness

Healing is excepting your past

Healing is letting go of the pain

Healing is letting others help you

Healing is listening to you

Healing is moving on past

Healing is a teardrop

Healing is a simple smile

Healing is a hug

Healing is a moment of time

A wonderful world

You cannot save the world single handed, but you can contribute.

Have positive thoughts every day.

Think how can I serve for the greater good.

Donate some time to a good cause.

Help Mother Earth and her environment.

Teach someone goodness today.

Listen to those around you.

Except each other's faults and forgive.

These are all simple thoughts and gestures.

Let them become part of your everyday lives and you will shine a light into dark corners of your world.

If we all did this every day imagine what a wonderful world it would become, we just need to unit and be as one.

Reach for the stars

Reach for the top of the highest mountain

Reach for the top of the highest trees

Reach beyond your wildest dreams

Reach into your heart for strength

Reach to your higher self for guidance

Never look down never look back, just reach for your dreams, they are within your grasp.

June

The first of June brings new blooms, hope and rays of sunshine.

Walk in Mother Nature and smell her healing scents.

Be transformed with her positive energies and vibration.

Let June heal you and bring a smile to your face.

Inner healing

Inner healing comes from within the soul.

Your heart is love; your mind can be the disease.

If you let your mind run in a negative thought pattern, your body will be dragged down with it.

When negative thoughts come in, hit them out the ballpark with a big bat in your head, and think of someone you love or a favourite moment in time.

Your body will start to fill up with positive energy, lifting your inner being. This then sends positive waves round your body healing it as it goes.

Heal from within.

Turn Dark into light

If you are feeling your days are dark
Pause…
Light a candle and make a wish
Listen…
We are all around you to give you strength
Feel…
Ask for a sign from us to be near
See…
It might be an angel feather
Touch…
We will touch your heart and inspire you
You…
You are loved and precious to us
Light…
Light your candle and shine into your world
Love…
Love is all around you, love yourself.

The magic of words
Fiction or Non-fiction

Fiction is a make believe existence.

A world of fantasy and make believe.

Non-fiction is truth and the real world.

Which do you live in, do you dream of a better world.

You can all make this a world a better place, which is an equal safe world.

Work as one not, against each other.

Start to today, take one step towards your fantasy world.

It will be come your reality.

The future is yours

You have a life path you follow.

You can all make this world as one.

You should help and support each other.

Not tear each other down.

Your thoughts make the future.

You need to radiate positive loving thoughts.

You need to stand up and set the example.

You need to be strong and brave.

Move forward and shine your light.

Your children are your future.

You need to listen to their innocent minds.

You need to let them change the world.

You need to show them the path of light, let the children shine, the future is theirs.

Join as one

You are all as one.

You live in divide.
Come together as one.
Be whole and true.
Love and see as one.
Be as one and shine.

Live hand in hand.
Walk side by side.
Learn from each other.
Teach each other.
Support each other.
Guide each other.

Your world will be as one.
Move forward as a whole.
Do not divide each other.
Only thoughts of love.
All knowing will be yours.
You will live as one.

Do not judge

Do not hurt those near to your heart.

Look at your actions and theirs.
Do not judge too quickly.
Look at them as a whole.

If you cannot be together.
Pull apart, but keep them in your heart.
Rise above the hurt and forgive.
Life is for living and being happy.

True love is smiles and happiness.
Being together even from a distance.
Help, guide and support each other.
Do no tear each other down.

Only you can evaluate your life.
Do you smile, and laugh together.
Trust and have faith in each other.
Hold this in your heart and love life.

Look in your deepest part of your soul.
Their lies the answers and the way forward.
Be happy, positive and true.
Life will bring what is right for you.

Eternity of love is yours

Eternity of love is what we all seek,
open your eyes as love is all around you

Mother Earth is love, feel it in the air,
walk your earth and breathe it in

Love is in your children's innocent eyes and
love is in your human heart

Your heart can break due to your love,
but love is a treasure to remember

Love all that is around you in your life and
look for the positive things in your world

Love is for Eternity you have it forever,
just open your heart to behold love.

True self

Your true self lies within you.
What's on the surface can be a false exterior.

Remember that when you judge people, not
all is revealed and as it seems.

To know their true self, dig below the surface.
There will be resistance from past fear & hurt.

Don't judge your fellow man and woman.
Always look within and find their true light.

Every human has this torch of love and light.
It just gets lost through fear of the unknown.

Don't judge help them shine their light
You will find their true value in time.

Today

Do not worry of what might be.
Be in the now and understand yourself.
You today are what matters.
Know your true self and values.
The rest will be there for the taking.
Your tomorrow will be your now.
Your now will be in the past.
Let go and be at peace with yourself.

Be kind to yourself

To be whole is to be honest with yourself.

Time distorts memories and trust.
The memory left is not what truly was.

To trust is based on true self-worth.
Move on forward do not look back.

Your memories are left back in time.
Your past will always be there with you.

Bring forward the love not the hurt.
Time is your healer and just trust in us.

Mother Earth

Life is like Mother Earth; you keep spinning round in time.

Both slowly changing and adapting to different situations, sustaining yourself, being nourished by food and air.

Listen to your own heartbeat, know your true self.

Listen to Mother Earth she is reaching out to you, there is a shift, she needs to heal, and you need to heal.

Find your inner light and let it light up the world.

Bring love and faith to the dark corners of life by speaking out, let others here your words.

Remember one act of kindness brightens up Mother Earth.

One less act of non-pollution helps cleanse her, Mother Earth sings her song, let her heal.

Angel love

As you wrap your arms around the one you love, the angels wrap their love around you.

We are the safe warm feeling of love and security, the safety net of life for when you tumble.

We are here to guide and help you on your path, ask and we will be there with you.

Have no doubt or fear as we are near, call out and we will answer your wishes.

Look for the answers around you in everyday life, feel are love and strength as we walk beside you.

As we wrap our wings of love around you, know you are always safe and loved by the angels.

Release this pain

Your world showers sadness down on you that mankind has made and reflects out to you.

Your inner spirit will cry with others pain and sorrow; you will shed and wipe away a silent tear too.

Release this pain from your hearts so you can see the light on your path to travel your journeys'.

Yes listen, feel, then send healing wishes to the suffering and spirits that have gone home.

Surround yourself with our loves protection and live your lives shining your love out to mankind.

A heavenly shield surrounds you to protect you as we wish you to shine my friends and be you.

Tide of time

Time slips over you like a wave, let it wash away your fears.

Let it gently sooth your soul and wipe away your tears.

Feel the gentle ripples on your skin, feel our touch on your face.

All will resolve in time dear friend, just take life at a timely pace.

As you drift on the tide of time, you will feel our love and kiss.

We will take away your pain, your heart will burst with bliss.

So my friends have faith in us, give over your heart to our light.

You will now shine in the world, your love has won the fight.

Guidance

Guidance is the key to happiness from:

Your first breathe

Your first smile

Your first steps

Your first words

Your first actions

Your first love

Your first values

Live your talk

Walk your talk

Be true to yourself

Take this forward in your life and teach others true love and guidance.

Your inner self

Discover your inner self, your whole being, yourself worth and true-life values.

Celebrate your strengths and success, cast out any self-doubts and negativity.

Do not let others pull you down, you know your truth and who you are.

Strive to gain all knowledge you can, about life, love and mother nature.

Your inner self wants to grow and learn, starting with being you and trusting yourself.

SHINE my friend.

A New day

Every day is a new day.

Today is a new day, time to re-group, time to focus.

Evaluate yourself, judge your actions, and find your values.

Now step forward, remember you are you, be number one for a day.

Be YOU

Your journeys intertwine, like a vine in a forest. Forever searching for the light above the darkness.

You will grow fresh shoots on you life's path. Branching out into new exciting adventures.

Keep growing towards the sunlight my friends. Except the changes your growth will bring you.

Trust in the intuition you feel and breathe. Believe your own self-worth and beauty.

You are now the great vine in the forest. You have reached for the stars and shine.

Be strong and true, just be YOU.

Scatter your love

Harness the love around you and take it into your heart.

Nourish this love so it grows and envelops you.

Then scatter your love like seeds out to your fellow man.

As they catch the seeds they will blossom and grow.

They will then share their love with the world.

The love seeds carried on the winds to unseen people.

As the light and love grows in the shadow of man.

The world will become one in the love and light.

Today is a new day

Today is a new day my friends.

Push forward with your lives and step away from the dark into the light.

Every day is a fresh start for you all to wipe the slate clean.

Cleanse your soul of any negativity and bring in only positive light.

Treasure those close to your hearts and let their love in.

Surround yourself with only love, then this lets you love in return.

Life is a gift my friends, unwrap it and live it to the full.

The Circle of life

Think my friends off your life's path from the first breath you take, until you take your last. It's not an ever-ending circle; there is a beginning and end while on earth.

Fill this circle of life with love, compassion, empathy, kindness and strength. Be one of life's inspirers, leaders and the best example humanity can offer.

You have to fill your own circle up with love, don't think others will do it for you my friends; this is your story and your path, live it.

As your circle grows, you will draw others into it with love and kindness. It's does not matter how big your circle gets as long as it is pure of heart and filled with true values.

So my friends live your life to the full, let your circle expand to touch other hearts and inspire them from your sprit within.

Nurture your spirit within

Nurturing your spirit within is key to you travelling towards a life of light and love. Kindness, compassion, and empathy are just a few things that nurture the spirit within. Giving out love and receiving love back into your lives is also a key factor. Live in the positive energy Mother Earth gives you lifting your vibrations towards us.

All these will ignite your spirit, and your minds thinking. Don't be afraid to speak out your thoughts, passions and creative ideas. Think out of the box my friends and share these thoughts with the world and do not let your fellow mankind hold you back.

Now ignite your spirit within and shine into the dark parts of your world bringing love and light.

Your Ego

Your ego is like orange peel wrapped round you.

If you let the orange stay whole you never get to taste the juicy fruit of life.

Learn my friends to peel back the ego and take a bite of the offerings of creation.

Once you master this the universe and all it has to offer is yours.

So take the fruits of life my friends and leave the peel behind.

Change

To make the changes you seek lies within you.

Your human essence mixed with the spirit within is the strength you need.

Connect to us my friends, we are here waiting to help you on your life's path.

You have free will so the choice is yours

The breath of the wind

The journey of life moves along on the breathe of the wind. Leaves will tumble down before you on your path.

The question is my friends do you kick them away? OR do you stand, observe, admire and hold this gift from nature?

To stand and observe what's around you can become quiet space. You will recharge and set your minds thoughts on the right path.

Please watch where you tread in life like footprints in the sand. Once past, the sea will wash them away, the moment is gone.

Don't look back my friends always forward on your paths. Watch for the beauty of what we set before you, signs from nature.

The choice is always yours where you tread and the path you take. Take that moment in time to hold that autumn leaf and be still.

Find your destiny

Whispers of time float around your minds, like the soft gentle wispy clouds floating on a summer breeze. They just float happily, drifting, waiting for the day they are called up on.

When you learn my friends to settle your minds, you will be able to hold out your hands in front you and gently grasp these whispers from the past.

The softness of them will surround you holding you safe and gently nudging you in the right direction.

These whispers of time are your future; the wisdom they hold is what you have lost. Find this wisdom my friends so you can fulfill your destinies.

Heaven's flower

My dear loved one, you will always be within our hearts, as you fly back home with the angels to the gardens of heaven.

You will shine amongst the flowers, the heavenly blue skies, and the pureness and the love of the divine.

We search for your love; we search for your presence to feel your hugs again, knowing that one day we will meet at the heavenly gate.

You are wrapped round our hearts with love, never forgotten, knowing you fly high amongst the angels.

Find your place in the heavenly blooms amongst the stars, so you can shine down on your loved ones.

When we feel low and our hearts grieve, we will look to the sky seeking your smile to release the pain that arises within.

Our Angel

Why the loss of one so young, we hear people say? Why can they not live their life in full until they are old and grey?

Only heaven knows the answers to these questions, my friends, why they have taken one so young back into their angel wings.

Rest in peace, young spirit soul, and we have ease knowing that you are now whole, playing up in the clouds, having fun and running in the heavenly sun.

Our hearts grieve for you, my precious one, but we know a new life for you has just begun. We know not why you had to go home, all we know is you will never be alone.

We miss your physical presence and embrace, but we know you now sit in heaven's grace, and one day when we travel back home we will be reunited in the name of love, never to be broken or separated again.

Our hearts will always be as one, beating the same tune of love from heaven above. So rest in peace in the arms of the angels, my sweet one, and we wait for that day we meet again in heaven's realm.

Love and be loved

You are here to fulfil a role while on earth; you could be a teacher, shop assistant, father, mother, auntie, friend, doctor, scientist, explorer, leader, inspirer – these are just a few of them.

BUT your real purpose is to love and be loved, united in peace and living as one.

To help this, start by taking away the words *they, them* and *others,* and live in a single clarity of oneness.

The beauty of the morning

As the beauty of the morning dawns on yet another day, your world responds like a flower opening up its petals to the morning warmth of the rays of the sun.

Your spirit is ready for this next day, the next step on its path on this journey, while walking along in the warmth and the light that the sun gives your Mother Earth.

Enjoy the beauty, my friends, enjoy the song of nature, look into the depths of your oceans, as there is beauty hidden everywhere on your planet.

But take yourself also to the dark parts of your world where there are depths of despair still, and pollution that is hidden from the human eye.

These parts of the world have not yet found the beauty and the light that opens like a flower every morning that responds to the sun and lives its life as it should.

You can all help with prayer, positive thoughts, good will, love and acts of kindness to change the world you are living in.

Would it not be a wonderful thing for every human being to wake up and see the beauty of the morning, not knowing any fear or dread of the day ahead, and to only ever experience love and kindness?

All humans would then be embraced with love and light and be able to fulfill your lives to their best potential, giving and receiving so much love; imagine what your world could be like, my friends.

Imagine the beauty of the morning every day, every minute of your day, every second of your day, that feeling of wonder as you take in that morning breath of freshness of the earth's dew.

So we say to you, my friends, take these thoughts and spread love and light out into your world to every human being, and see the beauty that lies within mankind.

The raindrop

Water is the transparency of life, reflecting all it sees in its inner self.

The strength you seek lies within this life-giving force of nature.

The power of the wave that can knock you off balance in body.

The serenity of stillness reflecting the blue sky calms your mind.

A single drop of this life-giving force starts new beginnings for all.

One drop reflecting its world around you; look inside this power.

This drop has no foes, only knows the divine life force from above.

Touch the raindrop, absorb its pureness of energy, and reflect.

The single drop is part of a large universal force calling you to watch.

Stand out in the rain and be cleansed as it cleanses Mother Earth.

The single raindrop reflects you, your body and inner spirit.

Both are mirrors of the divine love and light you hold in your heart.

Mother Earth's sparkle

The earth dew glitters in the morning rising sun, as Mother Earth is frozen in time. The stillness of her seeps into your inner spirit, knowing Mother Earth is the provider for all human life.

As you walk along Mother Earth's path, you feel the crunch beneath your feet and the ice of her core. She freezes with the winter nights; she thaws again in the winter sun to give life.

She always awakens with the rising sun to beam out again into the universe of love. Her blue oceans shine like jewels out to all that look down on her. She is beauty held within the palm of a mass source of love.

So remember as you walk along Mother Earth's path in the morning frost of the dawn, Mother Earth is shining out into the darkness of space to bring hope to all of those who look up on her, as well as those on Mother Earth.

The hamster wheel

We know some of you have been feeling that life is over-running you at times, your minds going ten to the dozen, sleep being less than what it should be.

Thoughts like, you need more hours in the day, panicking at what lies ahead that week, too much to do or not enough to do.

We have the solution, my friends: you create your own worry and panics. Trust that all will be achieved and if not, does it really matter if something is left out or missed? After all, there is always the next day, next week, or next year.

We are all working with you, helping you set your spiritual targets, and you are all working well on this path. Some of you will achieve this quicker than others. Remember that this is because you still need to learn, there are lessons set in place you have yet to experience. Then you take the next step on your spiritual journey.

Your day-to-day lives, work, home play, relationships, are all part of this great plan you have set yourself.

So come off the hamster wheel, stop chasing your own tail, slow down, sit in the moment, reflect, plan, and prioritise. You need time to love, hug and be one with nature; make this part of your day. Slow down and enjoy your earth experiences; this will help with your spiritual path.

Jealousy

We would like to raise the subject of jealousy amongst humanity. Jealousy is a human trait we do not have in the spirit realm. We are very blessed to have eliminated this through our ascension over the millennia, as we eliminated fears and the type of mindset that creates jealousy within your human form.

Jealousy is part of your human survival instinct, my friends, just so you understand that it is a natural part of your make-up, a human trait. Your Ego is also there for human survival and protection, for mankind to survive in time of threat. If you did not have the divine spirit within, the ego and jealousy trait would be your only way of being. These human traits cloud your mind and stop you having clear ways of thinking.

Why do we say jealousy is for survival? If, for

example, you were trying to create a business so you could eat and pay your bills and you see someone else doing the same business better than you, this would create a jealousy within your human being. This often kick-starts the drive to do better, as you want to survive. Sometimes you not realise that this is lying within you, and actions you take are aimed at this person or the circumstances that create this feeling of jealousy. This can lie in your subconscious mind and trigger you to act in a negative away towards the person involved.

You might use words to try and stop them, causing friction, or you will let this feeling of jealousy eat you away inside. Anger can also build in you that you might not understand, and you lash out at those you love who are not involved in the situation that caused this upset, not really understanding why.

Key to recognising when you are being jealous is to know yourself, my friend, and the way you behave. When you feel jealousy building up inside toward someone, then put out a thought of love to that person or situation straightaway, and this will counteract the jealousy and the darkness that clouds your mind. You also need to analyse your feelings –

What is making you jealous?

Jealousy is also a trait that can help you improve yourself; as said earlier, it can kick-start your survival instincts, and push you to do better. Some of you have a stronger survival instinct and human drive than others. If we presented you all with the same situation in life, each one of you would handle it differently, and some would fail, some would succeed!

Jealousy can also be triggered through love. When you see a loved one receiving attention from another human, or they are more outgoing in their personality and seem happier than you, this can cause jealousy. You love that person but you cannot seem to keep up with them, or understand how they attract so many nice people, and always seem happy in their life, and you start to feel distant. There is love there from them, too, for you, but the jealousy seeps in and you let it take control of you; this is something humans must learn to change. You will do this when you accept other humans are different, and you are all on different life paths, this is the way of the human race, as you are all individuals. You will achieve and create at different times, and then you will change.

Once you accept this, you can then improve your life in a kind, loving way with no jealousy towards others, only love, support and kindness. When you ascend to this way of thinking you will be amazed at how you will achieve great things, because only a positive outcome will come your way.

The Christmas Gift

As Christmas approaches you see no light, the Christmas star is not so bright.

You are rushing around, wondering where the Christmas joy is to be found.

Your thoughts are with the past and present, missing the loved ones that have been Heaven Sent.

You wonder what the future will hold, and when your heart will feel whole.

The Christmas future is bright within you and the light will shine again.

The love you held for loved ones passed sits within the heavenly feast.

They await for your Christmas table to be laid, and family to gather in the joy of the day.

They will come in their turn to give you the wishes and hugs you yearn.

Watch out for the Christmas tingles and the soft brushed kiss sensation on the cheek, these are gifts from your loved ones in the heavenly seat.

Do not mourn us – we still shine bright like the star on Christmas night.

We twinkle like your tree lights do, shining brightly out to you.

We are the message in your Christmas cracker, bringing joy and laughter.

We are the loved ones forever after.

So hold a candle up to us, my friends, and wish us well in our heavenly realm, for we wish you well on earth too, as you celebrate a Christmas new.

Have a magical Happy New Year

Happy New Year to one and all, may your New Year start with some fun.

Don't look back, my friends, look forward with TRUST.

Don't look back, my friends, look forward with LOVE.

Tread your journey in the light as you were born to live, with love, kindness and honesty.

Believe in yourself and believe in us, and you will not waver from your life's path.

Do not rush into the New Year because of fear at what you might not achieve.

Take it day-by-day, step-by-step, and believe in the magic you can create.

Look into yourself and heal; give over the grief, anger and the pain you hold within.

Leave this with us, my friends, so you can move on into a better space.

When you have released this into the universe, your New Year will be filled with grace. You will see how it unfolds, enveloping you in our heavenly hugs.

We will protect you and move you forward, just trust we are by your side. We are always listening, we hear your thoughts, we hear your prayers; just trust the answers will appear.

Stay positive in the light, move out of the darkness and the shadows, because you have the right to see the divine, and the love that can touch you in this lifetime.

Watch for signs from the heavenly ones, trust they are from us, ask and you will receive.

Never doubt, my friends; always trust and you will have the most magical New Year.

Heal Mother Earth

We walk the paths of earth to enjoy the Mother Earth's Realm, to take in the sights and sounds of nature. But our hearts break when we see the human waste that clutters up the streams, a sight we do not like.

Nature tries to survive around the hidden pollution of man that lies within. The plastic bags that hide in the darkness slowly decaying, so many are hidden from view.

Your Mother Earth is trying to adapt but is getting lost within her soul, so please, we beseech you to look within your hearts and cleanse Mother Earth of Man's pollution, so she sparkles from within again.

We wish you to walk the paths of Mother Earth, enjoying her abundance and beauty without seeing mankind's pollution taking away this wish.

We want you to all be aware of what occurs day-to-day, the pollution in earth's waters, the beaches that are covered with the plastic of Man that's slowly choking Mother Earth.

This was never part of her plan. What else can we say but to ask all of you to stop every day and take note of the world around you. Pick up the pollution, pick up the waste, talk to others and encourage them, so the world can be cleansed and renewed.

Mother Earth wants nature to sing its best song, not to slowly die from the germs and pollutants of mankind. So, my friends, please love your world around you, protect, walk and enjoy mother nature so she can be healed and renewed, feeling healthy, loved and singing from her soul again.

Imagine

Imagine the world's currency is love

Imagine the world living in peace

Imagine everyone feels safe

Imagine only kindness

Imagine neighbours helping neighbours

Imagine going beyond the stars

Imagine infinite knowledge

Imagine abundance of health

Imagine Utopia on earth

Know the Spirit within

The magic of the sunrise

As the sun rises in the stillness of the morn Mother Earth takes a breath of the divine.

The light shining across the lands, awaking all life old and to be born.

The silence is awakened by the light beams, the chorus of life sings out again to you.

The stillness now has movement and a voice, your heart is awakened to Mother Earth's tune.

As the sun rises into the protection of the earth, your spirit stretches out to feel its warmth.

Your body absorbs its life-giving energy, you find your path and life's worth.

As the sun sinks slowly below the horizon the silence falls again on your spirit within.

Know, my friends, you can hear our voice and in the silence there is love held frozen.

Sit in the silence and listen, hear the night sound of the universe.

Connect to the divine light beams and you will shine, sparkle and glisten.

Section 4
Daily guidance messages for you

There is a lot of inspiration writings in the world which can be over whelming for some people who struggle with words, so we wanted to write a clear basic message to you all. This section will help and guide you with our simple messages working alongside your day-to-day life.

Please remember you all have a guidance spirit team working with you, ask them to guide you to the message you need today. Call upon your guides, they are there to help you. Mankind has free will, so that is why you have to ask us, we will then send guidance down to you. Watch out for messages and signs from us in your busy day-to-day life's.

Allow your inner light to shine

Knowing

Your knowledge grows on your life's journey. But you put up a barrier to obtaining this knowledge when you are negative and don't understand your own value and purpose.

When you lift in to a positive way of being, our knowledge and messages are there for you to read and learn from.

You will be amazed how the universe will open up to you and lead you to *'Just Being You'*, be confident in your own energy space and your lights will shine.

Make a wish

You make wishes every day, as you dream of better things in your life, or the lives of others. Make your wishes with true and good intent and the universe will hear you.

Don't worry about over-filling your wish pot, you can never have too many. But be patient as wishes will be granted when they are right for you on your life's journey.

Your future is full of granted wishes, it will take time, but your wish pot will slowly empty and become reality.

So take the time to make a wish today and the universe will hear you.

Be Inspired

Does the world around you inspire you?

Are you inspired by just being you?

What do you seek? You need to be inspired to seek your dreams.

Visit places that inspire you, breathe in the history of your world or other people's creations.

Take a walk in nature, observe and delight in mother earth.

Imagine your dream is your reality, search for inspiration and we will inspire your soul and create your dreams.

Forgiveness

Forgiveness comes from the heart and soul.

Don't hold yourself back on your life's journey by holding on to emotions that give you negative energy in your inner being.

Release these feelings to the universe, lighten your burden and as you forgive you make space in your heart and soul for new beginnings.

Positive energy will now fill your inner being, you will find it easier to forgive in the future.

Others will see your forgiveness and shining light and follow your example, the world becoming a happier place.

Your inner child

Your inner child lies with your spirit within and its higher self. When your inner child plays, sings and laughs then you are at peace and your spirit is lifted.

With the busy world you all live in this is sometimes suppressed and you feel left lonely, waiting for a friend to knock and ask your inner child to come out and play.

This is such an important part of who you are - your personality, vibrancy and sparkle.

So take time to play, skip, run and have fun, be with loved ones and your spirit will shine, smile, laugh and be happy.

Sparkle

Challenges

From the moment your spirit enters this world your life will be full of challenges.

Every challenge you face will help define you as a person and deepen your strength of character.

Draw on your inner strength to face these challenges. You will find this within your heart and inner being.

As you rise to each challenge in your life, you will find strength, confidence and wisdom.

You are the challenge, you have what you need, reach inside for your strength, rise above any fears and shine.

Reach for the Stars

Happiness keeps you resonating and your vibration strong and bright like the stars.

Your life will be faced with challenges that will knock you away from this place you all seek.

Obstacles are placed in your way on your life's path to challenge you. You will become stronger from these and this will enable you to reach inside for your inner strength to achieve happiness.

Allow yourself to be happy, you deserve this within your life. Look up at the stars when in doubt and feel their vibration resonating within your spirit within.

Reach for the stars and be happy

Honesty

Honesty comes from within the heart. You all seek this from those around you.

Wake up each day and say "I will give honest answers from my heart and seek honesty from those around me."

Honesty brings honesty. It will inspire you to travel your path with this value in your heart.

Teach this to the children in your life so humanity can carry this value down the generations.

Honesty will bring truth, be true to yourself and live from your heart.

Be true to yourself

Look into your inner being, it is pure spirit. Being true to yourself and others helps our souls stay good and true.

Being true to yourself needs you to take time to reflect and look around you. *Are you happy?*

You might worry about making the necessary changes to your life and how it will affect others.

When you are true to yourself and happy, then others around you will be happier. You will attract the right people into your life and your spirit will feel lifted and energised.

Stay true to yourself, this will help you with your inner being, which needs to shine and be happy.

Protection

When you are feeling vulnerable and exposed to negative energies from those around you, call on Archangel Michael for protection.

He will place you in a blue light that will surround you for as long as you need it.

Ask Michael to walk beside you, for strength and guidance. Give over to him the situations that are causing your self-esteem to be low.

When protected and feeling stronger, you will see the situations that cause you concern resolve and your energies will lift drawing more positive things in to your life's path.

Stand back, invite in Archangel Michael and you will feel your life change - negative energies will leave your body drawing in new positive energies and new beginnings.

Footsteps in the sand

As you travel your life's path you create your own footprints in the sand. But take a look behind you - they have faded in the sand as the tide washes in.

Don't try and retrace your steps and live in the past. Accept the past, forgive, release any emotion and move on.

With release of past anger and forgiveness your future footsteps will be clear and crisp.

As you take these new footsteps, learn to forgive as you move forward so you don't look back and try to retrace your steps as they won't be there.

Time has washed your footprints away; they are just a memory that cannot hurt you.

Healing

We do not know time in our world, but humanity needs time to heal.

Healing cannot be rushed, so take the time you need. Do not let others rush you. Only you will know when you are healed enough to step forward again in your life's journey and smile.

As you heal, you will carry on with your day-to-day life. Make sure part of this journey is communication, holistic healing and time out for yourself.

Your heart will lighten and every day will become easier. Look in the mirror smile and love yourself. Do not feel guilty for being happy again.

Your loved ones on earth and in spirit want you to be happy.

Animal kingdom

You are a lover of the animal kingdom and feel broken-hearted when you see the ill treatment of animals on earth.

Your animals resonate with your spirit within, your pets are your guardian angels on earth sent to look over you.

If you have not already, you will give many animals a happy, loving home.

Don't be afraid to give your heart to a pet because of past loss. They will always be in your heart and over the rainbow bridge in heaven waiting to play again one day with you.

Enjoy, play and laugh with your pets and they will lift your spirit, keep you grounded and keep your heart young.

Enjoy and play

To be content and happy within yourself you need to enjoy your life more. Enjoy your surroundings, your friends, your family, your work and just being you.

If there is an area of your life you do not enjoy, don't blame others, sit back and take a look at yourself. You can change this situation - just ask us and we will guide you.

Part of enjoying your life is finding time to play; as you relax and become more positive, positive changes will happen for you.

Take time for yourself, or a hobby, or go out into mother nature, walking and breathing in her healing love.

When you play you lift your vibration, this will then help you make any positive changes that need to be made for you to enjoy your life to the full.

Gullible

Gullible is a term used in your society for those who have been taken in by another person, have over trusted them and been let down.

We know you have felt this in your life from the moment you understood the meaning of this word.

These lessons of broken trust are all part of your life's journey. If Gullible means you have trusted wrongly then let it be.

You must never give up on that trust in your life. In trust you will find, hope, love, guidance and happiness.

Look for the good in any situation where you have been let down, rise above the negative and trust will be a day-to-day part of your life.

Empathy

Empathy is with-in you all. If you all looked on situations in your lives with more empathy then you would have better understanding of others and find forgiveness.

When presented with a picture in front of you, ask why the artist painted it, why they would use those colours and subject, what are they trying to express to you. Use this technique on situations that present on your life's path; you will find you will start searching for answers and evaluate situations better.

When you live your life with empathy, answers will become clearer to you and you will better understand those around you.

This way of thinking will become second nature to you; just think of the artist's picture rather than judge without thinking.

Think with your heart

Listen

Take time in your busy life to sit in nature and listen to her song. Sit in a quiet meditative state and listen to your own heart and breath. Ask for guidance and hear our words of wisdom.

As you learn to slow down and focus, this will help you listen to others around you. At the moment, you think are listening but you are not.

Ask yourself: Are they sincere? Is there passion in their voice? Do they have honest intentions? Are they trying to guide and help you?

Don't let your pride stop you listening and accepting their help. Use your intuition to decide what advice and help to accept.

As you start to listen you will find your life will open up, opportunities will arise, and that missing spark will reignite.

Consequences

Consequences in your life start from the moment you take your first breath. People's actions and words affect you and your inner being.

You can be in the same situation as other people, but you will all respond differently, and your reaction will have consequences for those around you and the energy in the universe.

Think before you speak, as your words will affect others' feelings; some are more sensitive than others.

Look at how you behave in your day to day life.

Be the best you can, live your life to honest and true values, be positive, and any action you take will have positive consequences for others.

Actions and words cause consequences that ripple through the universe; live in love and light and be aware of your own being.

Passage of time

As you follow the passage of time a long your life's path, you will sometimes feel you are spiralling down a time tunnel, your life spinning out of control.

Reach out your hands to us and put on the brakes. It's at times like these you need to stop and evaluate your life and where you are in your life's journey. As you stop to evaluate, look around you, identify what's making your life unbalanced and spiralling out of control.

Write down what you want to achieve, what's stopping you and how you think you can improve this situation. Then give all these feelings over to the universe. We are listening.

Time will start flowing evenly again for you, lifting you into a positive place where you can achieve your life's purpose.

Remember - put on the brakes when the passage of time is spinning.

Passion

Your passion for life comes from within your spirit and heart.

Life is full of passion for your lover, for creativity where your talents shine through, for reading, writing, nature, your job, your children, family, pets and life.

It is key to follow these passions in your life to get the best from yourself. When you achieve this you can then give your best to others around you.

Listen to your heart and see how you feel when you follow your passion in life. Your vibration is uplifted, your higher self resonates and shines.

Do not feel guilty about taking care of your own needs; when you shine, others around will too.

Follow the path of passion through your journey, find your inner self and shine out into the universe.

Compassion

To be human is to feel compassion. You witness this daily in your lives around each other and in the animal kingdom.

Your heart stops and flutters at the violence and suffering in the world. Your inner being is deeply saddened by what you can witness on modern technology.

A simple gesture, reaching out your hand to a fallen friend, or holding them tight as they grieve in your arms is compassion. Saving a bee that's fallen into a pond or helping those less fortunate than yourselves is compassion.

If there is a time in your life when you need compassion, please accept it with grace, as this is a gift to help you heal on your life's path.

Be compassionate in your day-to-day life and this will help you with the understanding of your human journey on Earth.

Wisdom

Your inner wisdom comes from centuries of knowledge across the universe. It is in each and every one of you, you just need to reach inside to find it.

As your life path grows you gain wisdom from knowledge, learning, making your own decisions, your worlds' spiritualists teachers and your history.

From the moment you take a breath you make decisions; some will be mistakes, think of these as experiences you can learn from to make wiser decisions in your future.

As you grow older, you then become the teacher passing this wisdom on to the younger generation in your life.

Live your life in wisdom as this is key to a brighter future for you, your wisdom will pave the way for enlightenment and miracles in your life.

Walk a path full of wisdom and shine your light into the darkness.

Life's Journey

The first beat of your heart starts this life's journey.

Your path has been mapped out for you and as you take your first breath your journey begins. You will have guides and guardian angels with you at all times to guide and help you.

We are listening and watching all the time; tune in to us to ask for help and guidance, we will answer and give you signs. This will be through written literature, your media, a new person in your life, thoughts and ideas in your head.

You have free will and it is your choice whether or not to accept the guidance given. Remember we will always give our full attention and love to any thought and help you ask for, with the intention of helping you along the best life's journey.

You are here to learn and inspire your higher-self, so enjoy this journey and let us walk along the path with you.

Your path

Continue on your existing life's path as all will become clear to you in the near future.

You have felt that you have been branching off one way then another, this is not a test from us, it is just where you are now in your life's journey.

There are path signs placed along the way but you are not aware they are there. Ask us for guidance and help on making these decisions. We will deliver signs to you over the next couple of days, but you need to watch out for these, so keep us in your thoughts.

Sit in your own space with no distractions, feel your inner being, give your questions over to us on these decisions you have to make.

You will know with your inner intuition when you see the signs. Your path will then be clear to move forward without worry, but please look for the signposts of guidance for future decisions.

Push through the mist

At the moment you are looking at the horizon and seeing a mist, and as you move forward this mist is not clearing. You feel as if you are waiting for a change in the wind direction then all will be clear. But the air is stagnant and the mist is thick.

You are what will make this change, so look inside yourself and ask, what are your greatest strengths? When you recognise them, question yourself. Are you using them to the fullest you can in your life?

Are you in the right job or relationship, where these strengths and talents can shine?

Once you see clearly the wind will change direction and the mists will clear. Once again there will be sunshine in your life, and others will smile at your happiness and new inner strength.

Ask your guides and angels to help with this transition in your life, we shower you with love and are listening.

Mind and body

Call upon Archangel Raphael to walk beside you daily to heal your mind and body.

When you are in physical pain or mental anguish ask for signs of how you can help yourself in your life to take the pain and worry away.

You need to re-access yourself and environment. Is it right and healthy for you? When you know the areas that need improving, ask us to help you to take action to improve your life.

Rest your body as much as you can and in a quiet meditative state ask for healing and guidance from Archangel Raphael.

When you see others suffering you can also call upon him to help and guide them too.

We will give you the strength you need. The angels want to help and spread our love, you are worthy of our help, so ask, we will be there walking beside you giving you the best quality of life.

Consideration

From the moment you understood your language you have been asked to consider others. It can be perceived as a selfish act when you do not consider others feelings and situations.

How do you feel when someone in your life does not consider your feelings or even your opinion?

Take time to step back and look at the people around you, imagine being in their shoes, what they are feeling and going through at that point in time. This is consideration.

Live your life considering others and ask to be treated in the same way. You will become a better person, have more understanding and your fellow humans will learn from your considerate ways.

Teach this to your children and your grandchildren so the world is a better place for them to grow up in.

Trust in the stars

From time of old mankind has used the stars to guide them on their journeys, sailing the vast seas, climbing the highest mountains. No challenge was too much for them as they trusted that the stars would guide them.

What direction are you going in at the moment-and who is guiding you?

You all have a compass of life, you feel it is spinning and it needs to stop on a point of guidance. Just stop and look around you. Are you happy? Is there someone who is knocking you off course?

On a clear night look up at the stars, reflect on this and ask the universe for guidance. We are watching and listening.

Be brave and take that next journey on your map, don't try and sail the world in one day, take it port by port; listen to your inner self and trust in the stars, as we are giving you guidance.

Lift your energy

For you to function well and be at your very best it is important your body energy levels are at their highest.

You need to look after your physical body better by making sure you eat a healthy, balanced diet. Research high energy giving food if you are very active. Daily exercise is very important for you - this will lift your mood, helping to bring stress levels down and bringing in more positive energy.

It is also important your inner spirit is energised too; you can achieve this with healing, meditation and grounding yourself. Also make time to do something in your life you love doing.

With a combination of the above you will be a new you. You will be lifted to a higher energy vibration, feel focused and be amazed at what you can achieve.

You are energy and you need to be at your best levels to achieve the best for yourself and for those around you.

The world as one

You are all from one source and if you all worked together as one in love and light, what a wonderful, peaceful world you would live in.

You are all spiritual and healers and as you take up this journey you will heal yourself and then teach this to others. Only you yourselves are holding mankind back, the part of you that does not believe or trust in us.

Connect with your inner being and higher self and when you feel comfortable with this and know yourself, take the leap of faith and learn; you all have a life's mission to fulfil.

We will guide you on your path on this journey and work with you to develop your skills, but you must work hard and ask us for guidance. Confidence and trust comes hand in hand. Look in the mirror and say, *"I can do this,"* and trust us, we will not let you down, we are here to teach you.

Our knowledge, love and inspiration is yours, trust and the rest will follow.

Message of love

Love is in you, it is in your inner being, your heart and all around you in mother earth.

We want you to feel this love, absorb its wonderful energy to lift your vibration.

You have so much love to give, just let it flow, don't let your past hold you back, you have enough love for everyone in your life and they need to see it.

As you give your love, accept love back into your heart, this will create the balance you need in mind and soul to be you.

Love your life; if you are not balanced in mind and soul then take time to reflect and make changes to help with this love transition.

The universe's energy is love, the basis of life is love, we shine our love down onto you, feel our love's warm glow and shine love out onto your world and the universe.

Communication

Your voice is not being heard at the moment by the people near and dear to you.

Tell them how you are feeling, let out any emotion that might arise with this communication.

Talking to each other is so important in your busy life's. If you do not do this the negativity and worry will build up inside you. This needs to be released.

When you take the first step to make amends with a loved one or friend, do this face to face. Let them see your eyes and how you feel.

If you wait for others to break the silence you could be waiting a long time; it takes a strong person to make the first move.

Sing your tune to the world, let others hear your voice; you will only hear divine music all around you in your life as the communication flows.

Conquer the world

As you travel you life's path on earth you may feel you are a tiny insignificant dot and your self-worth is low. Remember my friend, all of you, no matter what race or religion, are all as important as each other and we are all from the same loving light and are as one.

Each one of you makes a change to your world, every action you take resonates in the world's energy and affects it. Make your life's actions positive and loving, and you will attract this back to you.

Imagine the small dot you see yourself as spreading out around the world; as you imagine this your energy and pride in your self-worth will grow.

You are you, you all are one, you all make a big difference and are loved and guided by us.

Connect with us and we will help your dot grow and conqueror the world.

Your Journey

You have an old soul and have travelled many life journeys with us. You know this in your heart.

You have a wise connection with the universe, and people are drawn to your wisdom and inner power.

You can be sensitive to others' feelings and know when they are not happy within their own lives.

You have a shining light that naturally wants to help others, but understand you will not be able to help everyone - sometimes they need to find their own path. Walk alongside them and be there if they need you.

You are spiritual and healing is strong within you. Make sure you keep yourself healed and energised on this journey then others will gain from your healing light and wisdom.

Take a step forward and connect with us, we will guide and inspire your journey.

Time to play

It is time for you to play and laugh my friend.

Lately you have been working hard and have not had much time for yourself, friends and family.

Your need to take yourself back to the innocence of childhood play, and find your inner child again.

This spark has been lost and when you reignite it your soul will lighten and you will feel so much more like you.

Take yourself off to a place where you can relax, find a beach and build sand castles, have a kick around with a ball, do a hobby you are passionate about; playtime is your time, enjoy and relax.

You will know when you have back your inner child again - you will be more relaxed, you will look at life through a clear window, everything will seem brighter, laughter will be there again and the sun will shine in your heart.

Be decisive

At the moment you are hesitating on your life's path. You are feeling indecisive about your future and what to do next.

You need to take control of your life, to shift the negative energy and move forward.

Hesitating is normal for mankind as it's a safety valve so you don't make mistakes. But you are afraid to take the next step in case it's the wrong one.

Have trust in your inner self feelings, ask yourself which is the right decision for you.

You need some confidence at this moment in time. Look in the mirror and see your reflection, connect and think, "I am strength and trust my own choices."

Intuition is a gift for you all, so when you are indecisive, connect to this and the answers you need will be felt in your heart.

Moving forward

It is time to move forward with your life. You are holding on to grief and hurt from you past.

The emotions you feel could be from losing a loved one, a friendship, a pet or even a way of life you enjoyed. You will experience grief, anger, sadness, but now you need to experience acceptance.

With any type of loss the worst thing is to hold all the pain inside in your heart; let it go, release it to the universe. If you need support, seek counselling or a listening ear. Distract yourself with new friendships and find a new passion in your life and don't be afraid to care again.

We are here, dear friends, to help you through this, ask us to support you along this journey to acceptance so you can step into your light again to shine and be loved.

We want to hear your laughter again

Laughter

Laughter is so good for and your spirit within. It lifts your vibration to where it should be so you can feel happy with your life.

When did you last have a really good laugh and enjoy yourself? You need to be surrounded by light hearted people and humour.

If there is no laughter in your life, you are at a stalemate point in your life's path. You need to look around you, shed the baggage that's dragging you down and step into the sunlight.

Say to yourself, I deserve laughter and happiness every day of my life and I will make this happen. Repeat this 3 times a day to yourself, you will be surprised how you will begin to smile again.

Lighten your inner being with laughter and smiles

Acknowledgement

You are all aware of the world around you, but there are areas in your life you are not acknowledging.

This could be a problem that you are not facing at work or home, a member of your family or a friend.

You are afraid of the consequences if you do face this area of your life and are trying to protect yourself from hurt.

You need to take this step forward, and deal with the situation, you will feel emotion, but once you acknowledge this pain and move through it, your whole world will become brighter.

We want your heart to be full of love again and your soul lighter. Do not carry the burden in your heart. Evaluate yourself, acknowledge the areas that need changing in your life and have faith in us, we are here to guide you.

Intervention

It is time we intervene in your life's path, you have gone off track and need to be steered back on to the correct path for your life's journey.

As you read the first 3 lines you know we are right and you now feel inner emotion. Let your feelings flow out, clear your negative vibes, take a deep breath and focus.

Step one: write down how you feel at this moment in time.

Step two: write down what you would like to be in your life and the positive way you want to feel.

Step three: how can you change your life's path?

Step four: what steps do YOU need to take to make this happen?

Step five: TRUST

Now you know what you need to do. Hand this all over to your guides and angels. Every day, read out loud the positive place where you want to be in life, and look for the help we offer as we work alongside you to make these changes happen.

Have faith in yourself

There are times in your life when you will feel as if you are being tested and tested over and over again, pushed to your furthest limitations. You lose faith in others around you and yourself.

Take yourself back to a memory where you were at your happiest, note what emotions and thoughts come into your head from this memory. This is where we want you to be in your life.

Yes, challenges are placed on your life's path to learn from, but if you get into a pattern of negative thinking you draw negativity back into your life. Have faith in yourself to change your life around. Start to reset your thought patterns, for every negative thought, replace it with a positive.

As you start to reset your brain to thinking this way, you will start to draw in positive energy and notice the world around you starts to become brighter. Your life's challenges will not be such a battle and you will overcome them. Believe in yourself.

Humble

Feeling humble is a lovely natural feeling for mankind. Recognising the fact you are feeling humble means you know good from bad, have a compassionate nature and great understanding.

You are a hard worker and help others. They see your qualities and admire you but you feel modest, you do not do these things for recognition and feel humbled when others admire you.

Take pride in what you do and achieve, you are all here for different reasons on your journeys. Take the recognition and build on the energy it provides. This is positive energy and you will thrive on it.

Do not change the way you are, your kindness radiates round you and helps others. Yes feel humble, we like this quality in you. Keep working and giving as you are, we are here to guide you and support your life's journey.

Conclusion

Conclusion to you means a final solution, the end of a journey, a problem solved. But conclusion is much more; it has depth, knowledge and lessons learned in its meaning.

When you feel something is concluded, you move on with your life, but what will help you strengthen is when you reflect on what led to this conclusion.

Is it concluded? Are there unsolved feelings you need to resolve? Is there more you or others could have done? Or it might be as simple as reflecting on happy times with family and friends, what you love about them and your memories. It is important when you reach the final conclusion, you have no unsaid feelings and you are confident with the outcome.

We do not want you to hold bad energy and feelings in your heart. That is why it is important to take time to evaluate when you feel something is concluded. This will help you develop, and as you start to do this it will become second nature.

Learn with every conclusion in your live

Notes and inspiration

We have included these blank pages for you to record your own positive thoughts and inspiration my friends. They will serve you well on your life's path.

The magic of words

Notes and inspiration

Notes and inspiration

Notes and inspiration

Notes and inspiration

Notes and inspiration

Notes and inspiration

Notes and inspiration

Notes and inspiration

The magic of words

Notes and inspiration

Notes and inspiration

Notes and inspiration

Notes and inspiration

Notes and inspiration

Notes and inspiration

Notes and inspiration

Notes and inspiration

The magic of words

Notes and inspiration

Notes and inspiration

About the Author

Sharon from Bengalrose Healing is a medium, author, holistic healer, spiritual teacher and mentor based in the United Kingdom. *'The Magic of Words'* is part of a collection of books she has written. 'Utopia', *'The Magic of Spirit'*, 'Ayderline the Spirit Within', *'Step into the Mind of a Medium'*, 'Heavenly Guidance', *'The light within Atlantis'*, 'Your daily spiritual guidance diary', *'New Earth - The light beyond the horizon'* and 'Inspiration Guidance Cards'.

Sharon is also the founder of the 'One Spiritual Movement' community
www.onespiritualmovement.com
Facebook one spiritual movement

Sharon's books are available on Amazon and on her own website: www.bengalrose.co.uk.

Visit her website **www.bengalrose.co.uk** to find out more about Sharon and what she offers.

You can also find her on twitter @SBengalrose and
FaceBook Bengalrosehealing.

Sharon has a YouTube channel with over one hundred fifty spiritual guidance videos. Search

'Sharon Bengalrose'.

Sharon also welcomes contact through email: Sharon@bengalrose.co.uk

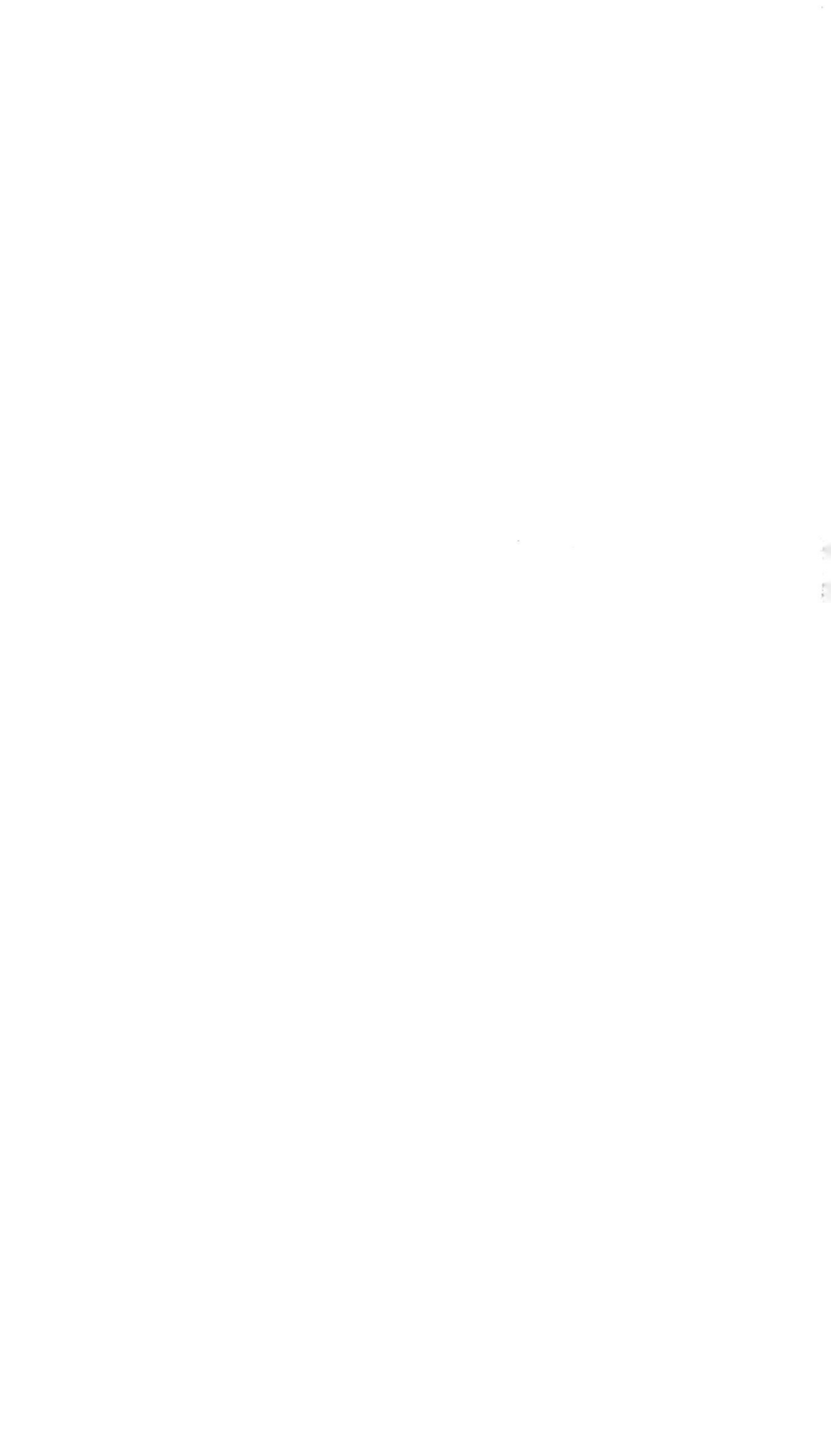